Personal Training Online

The Strategies to Successfully Produce Wealth When Teaching Fitness Anywhere in the World

Table of Contents

Introduction

As more and more people are becoming unfit and obese, more and more opportunities are opening up for personal fitness trainers or those who want to become one. But as an oriental perspective says, opportunities are disguised under challenges and problems. As such, personal fitness trainers need to identify and overcome certain challenges that come with the territory in order to become wealthy.

In this book, I'll identify those challenges for you so that you'll be able to prepare yourself for the work that's cut out for you. But more than just identifying those challenges, I will show you several strategies that you can use to overcome those challenges and achieve financial success in the personal fitness training industry. By the end of this book, you'll be in a very good position to start your personal fitness training journey towards financial success.

Are you ready? If so, turn the page and let's begin!

Chapter 1: The Challenges of Being a Personal Fitness Trainer

While being a personal fitness trainer is one of the most fulfilling professions in the world, it's certainly no cakewalk. So if you want to be a successful and rich personal fitness trainer, you'll need to be aware of these challenges. As I enlighten your mind concerning these challenges, I want you to keep in mind that the purpose of me doing so isn't to discourage you from pursuing or continuing to pursue a career in personal fitness training but to give you the opportunity to prepare for this comprehensively. You can only defeat the enemies that you know and your chances of defeating them are much, much higher when you prepare for them even before you face them.

Physical Resources

Unless you're a calisthenics kind of guy, you will need equipment – lots of it – and a place to house such equipment. And more than just having a place to do so, that place must also be a very comfortable and safe one. Gone are the days when sweatshops were the norm for gyms.

Most trainers who are just starting out don't have enough financial resources to have their own equipment and gym. Putting up a very modest gym will definitely set you back tens of thousands of dollars at the very least. For most people, maybe you included, such an amount is akin to an arm and a leg - maybe both arms and legs even. That's why most physical trainers start their careers partnering with gyms, which leads me to another challenge for physical trainers.

Income Sharing

By virtue of the word "partner," personal fitness trainers who decide to partner with gyms in order to practice their professions end up sharing the professional fees they earn with their partners. And often times, the gym takes a big slice of the trainers' income pie and for good reason: they bear all the financial risk having invested in the physical resources needed for the trainers to be able to train people.

You may be thinking that the solution to this is to take on more clients to have more income, and you'd be right in thinking so! However, taking on more clients also leads to another kind of challenge.

Time

Personal fitness trainers can only take on one client at a time. Otherwise, it wouldn't be personal fitness training any more. It therefore makes a lot of sense to take on more personal fitness training sessions and commitments in order to get around the income-sharing conundrum and earn lots more money. But there's a catch: everybody gets 24 hours a day only, regardless of social status, occupation, age or gender. That means taking on more clients and sessions will reduce the amount of time you have for just about everything else.

This may not be a big concern for personal fitness trainers who are single, ready to mingle, and have no dependents and active social lives. But for personal fitness trainers who are already married, are in a serious relationship with a partner and have very young kids, this can be a very serious challenge. Unfortunately, it's one that has no workaround. It's either personal fitness trainers spend more time training more clients or allot enough time for other important areas of their lives. It's an either-or proposition.

Certification Requirements

Personal fitness trainers need to be certified by a reputable accreditation body, such as ACE in the United States, in order to get enough clients, particularly those who are willing to pay higher personal fitness training fees. More than just a requirement, official certifications act like a badge or seal of quality that tells clients that a particular trainer knows his or her stuff very, very well. It's basically like hiring an accountant for your business. You'd rather have someone who's a certified public accountant do your books rather than someone who isn't, right? Right!

But certifications aren't exactly cheap, whether financially or in terms of time. In order to get certified, a trainer will need to fork out serious cash, which is at least a thousand dollars for taking certification exams as well as for review or study materials that can be studied at the trainer's free time. But if the trainer wants to seriously increase his or her chances of passing a certification exam, enrolling in a review class may be needed. And that of course, costs money too.

Client Problems

Getting clients is a challenge for any given freelancing profession or entrepreneurial endeavor. And as more and more people are getting into personal fitness training, whether as a trainer or as a self-taught client, it becomes even more challenging to get clients and keep them. In this day and age, the ability to leverage the Internet –

especially social media – is a very crucial skill to learn.

But even after getting clients, personal fitness trainers' client-related challenges continue to persist, although in different forms. One of the challenges personal fitness trainers face is the need to adjust to the whims and wants of clients, particularly their schedules. If the client has a day job, it follows that he or she will be available for training after hours or on weekends only, which can be a personal fitness trainer's most important personal time. If the personal fitness trainer is newly married or has a new baby, adjusting to the clients' time may pose some challenges in their marital relationship.

Another challenge that clients can give their personal fitness trainers is attitude and one problematic attitude is pride. Some clients, especially those that are already experienced when it comes to physical training, can be quite difficult to coach simply because they feel they know better than their personal fitness trainers. Another attitude is skepticism coupled with negativity, always questioning the exercises or routines that trainers give them. Lastly, the tendency to just not do what the trainer says is another problematic attitude that can discourage personal fitness trainers because lack of results is often viewed as a personal fitness trainer's lack of skill or ability to produce results for their clients.

Trainers who aren't comfortable going after potential clients and succumbing to their every whim will find the marketing side of personal fitness training to be quite a challenge. Let's face it; personal fitness trainers more often than not need clients more than the clients need personal fitness trainers. And having to succumb to most of clients' wishes and requests is an inescapable part of personal fitness training and just about any other profession that provides services.

Another client-related challenge for personal fitness trainers has to do with collection of professional fees. Some clients are just plain thick-skinned and inconsiderate to the point that personal fitness trainers have to shed sweat, blood and tears just to collect their hard-earned fees. Some clients also quit altogether after finding the training sessions "too hard". The worst case scenario is when other personal fitness trainers steal other trainers' clients. After all, it's a dog-eat-dog world out there.

Losses and Burnout

To the extent that all the aforementioned challenges exist, personal fitness trainers may not make enough money for their needs or for going after their dreams. And I don't care what many people say about money, i.e., that money is the root of all evil. I disagree because it's the love of money that does that and not money itself. And I also don't agree that love for money always leads to evil. After all, everybody needs money to survive and live a good life. Many personal fitness trainers burn out when they fail to earn enough money from their craft. And when they do, there goes their dreams and their opportunities to live out their purpose.

Chapter 2: Personal Fitness Training Riches

Just because there are many challenges to the personal fitness training profession doesn't mean you can't earn great money from training people to become fit. When you look at challenges from a different perspective, you can see that challenges are opportunities to earn even more money. How?

The challenges we presented in Chapter 1 are hindrances to many personal fitness trainers' financial successes. As such, these serve as "filters" through which the really good personal fitness trainers are separated from mediocre and bad ones. Those who are able to pass through such filters find themselves in a league of their own with only a few players sharing the abundant financial opportunities that personal fitness training can provide.

So if you're wondering if it's possible to become rich in the personal fitness training business, to that I say "Heck yeah!" You just need to know several important things that aren't fitness training-related. Let's take a look at those important things now, shall we?

A Financial Perspective

The reason why most fitness trainers fail to sustain their passion and profession is because of myopic thinking. In particular, they're only trained in the art and science of physical fitness training. "Duh, what else does a trainer need to be skilled in to succeed as a personal fitness trainer?" you might ask. Well, a trainer also needs to wear another hat or have another mindset that can complement the personal fitness training one: a financial mindset or perspective.

Why is having a purely personal fitness training mindset a fatal mistake for personal fitness trainers who hope to stay long in the game? It's because everybody needs money regardless if a person's into the personal fitness training business or into the restaurant business. And to have more than enough money, one must be able to exercise his or her profession in ways that ensure more money's coming in than going out.

The reason I'm pointing this out to you is because with professions that involve a lot of passion, as is the case with personal fitness training, it's easy to get carried away by emotions and fall into the "the only thing that's important is doing what you love because the money will just follow" mentality. Even if – for the sake of argument – money does follow you all the time while doing what you love, it will never be enough if you don't know how to minimize your expenses, especially those that are related to your being a personal fitness trainer. Only when you have a financial or entrepreneurial mindset can you ensure that you're being an excellent personal fitness trainer translates into being a financially secure one.

The Cash Flow Quadrant

A very important principle that you should master when it comes to having a financial mindset in your personal fitness training business or profession is the Cash Flow Quadrant, which was created by bestselling personal finance author. Robert Kiyosaki – he of the Rich Dad, Poor Dad book fame. The quadrant represents 4 typical sources of income: employment, self-employment, businesses and investments.

Further, these 4 types can be classified as active or passive. Active income refers to income that requires you to put in a lot of time and effort. And under this type are the employment and self-employment quadrants. Passive income refers to income earned with minimal effort and time and under this type are businesses and investments.

Without getting into too much financial mumbo-jumbo, Robert Kiyosaki teaches that if you want to become and stay rich, you must prioritize the business and investment quadrants. Why? It's because they offer you the greatest leverage for your time and effort, i.e., you earn more for the same amount of time and effort. Let me explain.

When you put up a business, it will considered as an active source of income in the beginning (self-employment) because setting it up and building the necessary systems and market will require you to personally supervise, manage, and work on the business itself. But as time goes by and you're able to put up the necessary systems, train the needed people, and delegate key tasks and responsibilities for running the business to competent and trustworthy managers, you'll be able to start scaling back on your personal involvement in running your business to the point that you no longer participate in its daily management. At that point, you will no longer have to put in as much effort and time to earn from it. And that's what will eventually turn it into a passive source of income. With the amount of time and effort you'll be able to free up, you can put up more businesses and increase your income even more!

Now let's talk about investments. Investments mean allotting financial resources in financial securities or income-generating assets that will make you even more money. In other words, investing means making your money earn more money for you even while you sleep. When you invest in financial securities or income-generating assets, your only work or job is to carefully evaluate which financial securities or assets will you invest in. Once you've placed your money there, you'll just need to monitor it every now and then and just wait for money to arrive.

From Active to Passive, From Employment to Entrepreneurship

As a personal fitness trainer, your profession is considered an active income source either as an employee or a self-employed (freelance) trainer. Being such, your ability to exponentially increase your earnings is very limited because you will be limited by the number of hours you'll be able to work or train people, which in turn limits the number of clients you can serve at any given day. But if you can transition from merely being a personal fitness trainer to a personal fitness training entrepreneur, you can effectively multiply yourself and your income even as you reduce your working hours. By becoming a business owner or entrepreneur, you'll be able to trade in working hours for more dollars.

How can you make a business out of your personal fitness training profession and become wealthy? The key is to diversify or establish multiple streams of income that are tied to your personal fitness training services. What you'll need to do, which I'll show you in the remaining chapters, is to leverage on your personal fitness training expertise and build an international personal fitness training business using the power of the Internet.

Chapter 3: Personal Fitness Training Blogs

The easiest way to set yourself on your way to making a business out of your personal fitness training expertise is to start a personal fitness training blog. Yes, a blog!

You may support your protests to the idea with statements like "I'm not a writer" or "I can't write squat even if my life depended on it." Yes, there's a reason why you're a personal fitness trainer now instead of a freelance writer, blogger or social media expert. But here's the thing. You don't have to know how to write to have a blog. Heck, a lot of bloggers and self-published authors didn't even have a clue about how to write a blog or a book when they first started but were able to successfully put up their own blogs and even make money from them. How?

Outsourcing. Yes, many of them hire ghostwriters to write their blogs or books for them. But one thing you can't outsource are your ideas because you alone know your market and what types of content will attract them.

So how do you start blogging and how do you make money from your personal fitness training blogs?

How to Earn Money from Your Personal Fitness Training Blog

There are several ways you can earn money from your personal fitness training blogs. One of them is through advertisements. If you've ever clicked on advertisements on some of the websites you've been to in the past, you may remember being redirected to another website, usually the advertisers' home or landing pages. When you did that and were redirected, you allowed the owner of the website that featured the ad to earn money from what's called as pay-per-click advertising, i.e., advertising revenue from people who click on advertisements placed on websites. When you've put up a blog site and advertisers place advertisements on it, you can also earn money every time your blog site's visitors click on those advertisements.

The key to making money from advertisements on your blog site is pretty much the same as for television – you need to have enough visitors on a regular basis, i.e., subscribers, to which advertisers can show their ads. If your website's like a ghost town, don't expect advertisers to place ads on your blog site. So the key to getting ads placed on your blog site and earn money via pay-per-click advertising is to attract frequently returning visitors via great content.

As well, you can market your own or affiliate products. If you have a product or service you would like the world to know about a blog is a major way to get the word out. Just create an inexpensive banner ad that links to the product and strategically place it where most readers will see it. "Boom" extra advertisement for your business.

The same can be done for an affiliate product. Simple sign up at Clickbank.com, Jvzoo.com, or Commission Junction (cj.com). Once there you can find tons of products to market. When someone buys a product from your blog you get a commission. This is an extremely popular practice. And most people have no clue that hundreds of millionaires have been created this way. If done properly, affiliate marketing is one of the most powerful weapons in an personal fitness trainer online arsenal.

Another way to earn money from your blog site is through direct sponsorships or advertisements, where you get paid to feature an advertisers products on your blog site through product reviews or endorsements. In the example I've given earlier, there is a middleman or an intermediary between you and the advertising company or businesses itself – such as WordPress.com's WordAds program. In a direct sponsorship or advertisement, you and the advertiser directly communicate. As such, you get 100% of the advertising revenue from the client. As with pay-per-click advertising, a good amount of regularly occurring blog site traffic is needed to justify sponsorship of you blog site. For this purpose, the ability to consistently generate engaging content is a must.

Putting Up Your Blog Site

There are several ways to start a blog but what I will teach you here is the easiest and most convenient one – WordPress.com. This particular platform allows you to start a blog even if you have zero knowledge about website design and programming. All you need to know is how to navigate the web and you're on your way to putting up your very first blog in minutes.

Start by opening up a WordPress.com account in their website, which should be fairly easy if you know your way around the Internet. You have several types of accounts to choose from: free, personal, premium, and business plans. If you want to start earning right away through advertisements under their WordAds program, you'll need to open a premium or business account at the onset, which costs more than a personal plan. But if you're not in a hurry and can afford to gradually build up your blog sites traffic, you can start with a free or a personal plan and wait until your blog site has enough regular traffic to justify registration under the WordAds program.

More Advertisement Income

If you choose to put up your blog using WordPress.com, there's a tradeoff for the ease and speed at which you can start blogging: limited advertising income. In particular, your advertising income will only come from WordPress.com's WordAds program. If you want to enjoy advertising income from top sites like Google (via Google AdSense), Lijit, OpenX, Buy and Sell ads and Vibrant Media, you will need to sign up for a self-hosted WordPress account, which is WordPress.org. Because a self-hosted blog is much more difficult to set up and maintain for a beginner, I suggest you build up your blog site first under WordPress.com and, when it has grown to gigantic proportions, you can migrate to a self-hosted one under WordPress.org later on.

Chapter 4: Personal Fitness Training Videos

As mentioned earlier, you can only increase your personal fitness training income – whether as an employee or a self-employed person – by taking on more clients. We also mentioned earlier that it could prove to be especially challenging because there's only one of you and many of them out there. But if you make personal fitness training videos, you'll be able to effectively "multiply" yourself and train many people simultaneously anytime and anywhere. With training videos, you can train 100 people at the same time, even more! Imagine that!

There are 2 ways you can earn through your personal fitness training videos: YouTube ad revenues and product placements. Let's take a look at YouTube first.

YouTube Channel

When you put up your own personal fitness training channel, you can consider it as your video blogging site, which many people refer to these days as "vlogging"- a combination of the words video and blogging. As a type of video blogging site, you can also earn through advertisements when you "monetize" your videos on the platform. When people watch the advertisements played at the start of your personal fitness training videos, you can earn advertising money off that. So the key to making a lot of money from YouTube is to garner as many loyal viewers or subscribers as you can. Just consider your personal fitness training YouTube channel as another TV channel where the more viewers you have, the more advertising income you can earn.

As with your personal fitness training blog site, the key to earning good advertising revenue is to populate your YouTube channel with great and engaging content, i.e., informative, interesting, and entertaining personal fitness training videos. Nothing else will give you significant advertising revenue from your YouTube channel than that. As a general guideline, such videos should be:

- Generally short and concise, around 2 to 3 minutes tops;
- Packed with uniquely useful information, i.e., information that only you or only a

few other YouTube video creators can provide;

- Good quality videos, i.e., shot with a high definition or resolution camera, well-lit, clear and crisp audio; and
- Able to provide viewers with calls to action, i.e., subscribe to your channel, share and like the videos, etc.

Product Placements

When you've built a big enough subscriber list and have established yourself as an authority figure when it comes to personal fitness training and fitness, you can start looking for companies that would be willing to sponsor your YouTube channel or videos via direct product placements. The beautiful thing about this is that you get all the advertising revenue and don't have to split it with YouTube. This is a really great way to get rich!

So how can companies make direct product placements on your YouTube channel? One is through your product review videos. As the name implies, you create videos that review different products that are related to your personal fitness training niche such as supplements, apparel, equipment, programs, and even gyms. Of course, it goes without saying that you keep your reviews objective and shouldn't be biased towards the advertiser or product placer.

Another way you can profit from direct product placements is by creating videos that teach your viewers how to use certain products, programs, or services related to your niche. This is a great way to promote your sponsors' products and services because it gives your viewers the opportunity to see how a specific product or service can be used and if it's something that they can practically use. Most of the time, people are hesitant to buy products because they're afraid it'll be quite difficult to use or may not work for them. And by providing them with videos on how a specific product, service, or program works or can be used to help them achieve their personal fitness goals, you'll be able to help your sponsors increase their sales. And that my friend will help you successfully turn your personal fitness training profession into a personal fitness training business that'll give you passive income.

Chapter 5: Personal Fitness Training Products

Finally, you can transform your freelance or employed personal fitness training gig into a business endeavor and earn lots of passive income by creating your very own personal fitness training products that you can sell online or on a physical store. What are these products?

Personal Fitness Training Courses

If you have neither heard of Udemy.com nor visited their website yet, you should. Why? It's a great place to sell your very own personal fitness training video courses. Many people have already become millionaires by selling video courses on a multitude of topics from computer programming, Internet marketing, and even how to start a business. You can create just about any course on topics that you're really good at, such as personal fitness training, and upload it there so people who are dead serious on getting fit can buy your video courses and achieve their fitness goals.

Why not just sell those courses on your blog site or YouTube channel? One important reason why websites like Udemy should be your top priority – especially as a rookie entrepreneur and online marketer – is logistical convenience. You don't have to worry about putting systems in place on your website that will facilitate secure and convenient payment options because websites like Udemy will take care of that for you. And more than the payment mechanism, Udemy takes care of all your videos' hosting needs. Just upload your videos and people can start enrolling in your video courses.

Another important reason for prioritizing websites like Udemy is integrity. Unless you're an internationally known personal fitness trainer like Gunnar Nelson or – God forbid – Richard Simmons, you have your work cut out for you in terms of convincing your prospective customers that it's safe to fork out their precious dollars online to purchase your personal fitness training courses. But if you're courses are available on Udemy.com, then they know that you're not a huckster and that you actually have a product to sell.

E-Books and Other Downloadable Digital Materials

If you have a very effective personal fitness training program, you can make tons of moolah by coming up with your very own downloadable personal fitness training e-books, like what premiere personal fitness trainers like Tom Venuto (Burn The Fat, Feed The Muscle), Shaun Hadsall (The 4-Cycle Solution), and Jeff Cavaliere (Athlean-X) have done. These guys have created their own downloadable digital manuals and in so doing, have practically trained thousands of people and helped them get into the best shape of their lives without meeting them at all. Talk about multiplying themselves thousands of times all over the world and earning lots of money in the process!

Personal Fitness Products

From shirts, to accessories and supplements, you can leverage the power of the Internet through your very own blog site, social media and YouTube channel to sell your very own personal fitness merchandise. Some of the most successful people who've done this are retired famous bodybuilders like Rich Gaspari (Gaspari Nutrition), and Dorian Yates (Dorian Yates Nutrition). They leveraged on their physical fitness expertise and successfully launched their very own nutritional products. But the key here is to establish yourself as a reputable authority when it comes to personal fitness. And how can you do that even if you're not a celebrity fitness trainer of bodybuilder? That's right, by attracting a lot of followers on the Internet via your personal fitness training blog, social media page and YouTube channel by regularly generating great content that people will find very helpful and practical.

Chapter 6: Key Investments Needed

As we end this book, let me share with you how you can successfully create your personal fitness training empire using the strategies I've enumerated from Chapters 3 to 5 by investing in several important things.

A Very Good Ghostwriter or Ghostwriting Service Provider

Remember how I said earlier that you don't need to be a good writer in order to come up with a great personal fitness training blog or an excellent personal fitness training e-book or program? I meant that because with the advent of the Internet, it's very easy to find a ghostwriter who'll write blog posts or articles and e-books for you for a fee. You can go to websites such as The Writing Summit, UpWork.com (formerly oDesk.com) or Fiverr.com to hire ghostwriters who will write your blogs, articles and e-books for you.

But the responsibility of coming up with great content doesn't rest on the ghostwriters alone. You also have a part to play, particularly coming up with specific ideas for the materials they'll write and the overall theme of your posts and e-books. They will only be able to write what you specify and if you don't specify anything, don't expect them to read your mind and come up with an excellent product per your standards.

Make sure you also relay your instructions to them very well. If you don't, you'll run the risk of getting a well-written product that still won't be up to par with what you really have in mind. Ghostwriters aren't psychics so for your benefit, make sure your instructions are clear.

Good Quality Video and Audio Equipment

You don't need to spend tens of thousands of dollars for such equipment. A good DSLR camera with HD video capabilities or even a top of the line smart phone such as the iPhone and Samsung Galaxy have very good video capture capabilities, which will enable you to capture high definition personal fitness training videos. It will also be helpful if you can grab a good tripod so you can shoot stable videos.

When it comes to audio equipment, two of the best pieces of equipment to invest in are lapel mics and a portable audio recorder that you can clip clandestinely on your clothing. Using such equipment, especially if you're shooting an instructional video, minimizes background sounds and echoes, giving your videos excellent audio quality.

Powerful Computer and Good Video Editing Software

If you want to produce very good quality personal fitness training videos, you'll need to use a good video editing software, which requires a powerful computer to run smoothly. In my case, I use Apple's MacBook Pro and for software, I use a combination of iMovie, Camtasia, and Viddyoze. The MacBook's hardware is capable of handling iMovie and Camtasia smoothly. I use iMovie as my primary video editing software and I use Viddyoze – an online video production service – to create stunning intro, outro, logo, and transition video clips. I use Camtasia only for further enhancements on a few of the clips I've created using Viddyoze so that I can use them on iMovie. The beautiful thing about most powerful computers in the market today is that they normally come with good entry-level video editing software such as the Mac's iMovie or Windows' Movie Maker.

Market Research

Not all your investments involve shelling out serious money. Market research is one of those relatively cheap investments you can make that will allow you to come up with consistently great and engaging content for your personal fitness training blogs, YouTube channel, and downloadable digital products by giving you ideas of what your target market wants. And according to Internet marketing maverick Kelvin Dorsey, you'd be better off catering to what people want rather than what they need. I agree with him because what's the point of coming up with something people need if they don't want to buy it in the first place?

Investing in market research can be done easily and practically for free. How? Learn how to mine websites such as Reddit.com and Quora.com, where many people get together to ask questions about stuff they're very interested in. Questions are indicative of what people have in their minds or the things they want to address and these two websites will help you check out a lot of people's questions concerning personal fitness that can help you come up with spot-on personal fitness training content.

You can also use Google's Keyword Planner to discover the hottest personal-training keywords being searched as of the moment. Keywords are the means by which people search for answers in Google and Keyword Planner allows you to discover what many people are looking for via keywords. It gives you much needed stats like average number of monthly searches and how much advertisers are willing to pay to rank high in certain keywords. For a simpler tool, simply download the Keywords Everywhere extension app for Google Chrome, which can give you quick stats on keywords you want to search for on Google via its Chrome browser. Such stats include average monthly searches, cost per click for advertising using a particular keyword, and the level of competition for that keyword. Keyword Planner is free so get it now!

Conclusion

Thank you for buying this book. I hope that more than just helping you learn more about how you can become a wealthy personal fitness trainer wherever you are, it was also able to encourage you to take steps towards achieving your goal of becoming a financially successful trainer.

And that brings me to another important point that I haven't covered yet in the book: knowing is only half the battle to achieve your goals. The other half is action or application of knowledge. Therefore, I strongly encourage you to start acting on the things you learned here as soon as possible. The more you delay, the higher your risk for not doing anything at all becomes. And with that comes higher risks for not achieving your financial goals as a trainer.

You don't have to apply everything at once. The truth is, it's impossible. As with building muscles and getting fit, it starts with taking baby steps that gradually build up over time. Start with putting up your blog site first and take things from there, one at a time. Rome wasn't built in a day but they were laying bricks every hour, as the saying goes. So it is with your personal fitness training business empire – you build it one brick at a time.

Here's to your personal fitness training financial success my friend! Cheers!

If you want help to get started today creating your business online as a personal fitness trainer go to www.fitnessdollars.net today and down load my other book for FREE. The Problem With Modern Day Personal Fitness Training

Made in the USA
Middletown, DE
28 January 2018